SUMMARY OF

HOW TO CHANGE

YOUR MIND:

WHAT THE NEW SCIENCE OF PSYCHEDELICS TEACHES US ABOUT CONSCIOUSNESS, DYING, ADDICTION, DEPRESSION, AND TRANSCENDENCE

By
MICHAEL POLLAN

Brought to you by

Anthony Young

Table of Contents

GENERAL OVERVIEW

In *How to change your mind*, Michael Pollan traces the eventful history of psychedelics, from Hofmann's first encounter with LSD to the first surge of research into the field, to the widespread abuse and misuse followed by a federal government ban, and the recent resurrection of psychedelic research. Psychedelics are probably the world's most controversial class of drugs and in this book, he narrates how they got their reputation.

Pollan is careful to correct the popular conclusion that Timothy Leary was the beginning and end of psychedelics. The author's depth of research is obvious as he chronicles the lives and contributions of scientists, therapists, religious leaders, and countless others who have a place in the psychedelics story.

His description of psychedelic journeys traveled by people are interesting, especially the narration of his personal experiences.

Throughout the book, Pollan provides answers- *in the form of interviews with experts*- to many of the questions about psychedelics. One of the controversies that have plagued psychedelics from inception is whether it is therapeutic or mystical and Pollan does his best to place both on an even ground, leaving the answer to each individual.

CHAPTER 1: A Renaissance

Key Notes:

- *Events leading up to the resuscitation of psychedelic research culminated in the year 2006*
- *LSD's beginnings had nothing to do with spirituality*
- *Many researchers blame Timothy Leary for the initial banning of psychedelics*
- *Psychedelics are one of the most misrepresented drug classes*
- *The 2006 study of Griffiths, Jesse, and Richards paved the way for psychedelics' second chance*

Many are not aware but the incidents which heralded a turning point in psychedelic research date as far back as the year 2006. Interestingly, the three incidents were in no way related so it's no surprise that only a few could see a resemblance of connecting dots. The first incident occurred in Switzerland at the 100th birthday celebration of Albert Hofmann. To scientists, Hofmann was more than a human being. He was somewhat of a god. Back in 1938, Hofmann, who was then a chemist, discovered Lysergic acid diethylamide, a psychoactive molecule more commonly referred to as LSD. But it was not until 1943 that he would become aware of his discovery, and the story of how that happened is one that no one tires of hearing.

Hofmann was not the typical 100-year old. He was actively involved in the activities planned to mark his milestone birth anniversary and not surprisingly, the crowd gathered asked for a retelling of how he came about LSD. Hofmann told of how he discovered LSD-25 as a molecule in the fungus, Ergot. It is important to know that Ergot did not have the best of reputation. It was known to infect grain and subsequently cause a sort of insanity in those who consumed products from the same grain, but it was also useful for inducing labor and to stop bleeding in women who had just put to bed. The laboratory for which Hofmann worked as chemist knew this, hence, the task to find new drugs.

Hofmann isolated LSD-25 as he named it, but discarded it after testing did not reveal any significant effect on the animals. Interestingly, Hofmann did not discard LSD-25 as usual. Instead of tossing it out in the trash, he left it laying on the shelf. It wasn't until five years later- sometime during World War Two that Hofmann would be mysteriously drawn to the jar. He intended to re-investigate the molecule and proceeded to do just that. Somehow, his skin came in contact with the molecules and he began to experience weird sensations. His body felt strange and he seemed to be in a trance; transcending a new level of consciousness bursting with color. The fact that Hofmann's body came in contact with the LSD-25 was another mystery, seeing that Hofmann always went to great lengths to protect himself when handling poisonous chemicals. He did not know it at the time but what he experienced became the first of what is now commonly known as LSD- or acid- trip. To say the least, Hofmann was enthralled by his experience. It was like opening a door halfway and liking what you see. Your next step is likely to involve opening the door all the way. So Hofmann dissolved a very minute portion of LSD in water and drank it. This time, his experience was so out of this world that he was convinced of his own insanity. He thought he was going to die and had the doctor summoned. Hofmann was in strange realms. He was seeing well-known objects taking on bizarre shapes and moving. He himself was highly hysterical, but at the end of the day, the doctor found nothing wrong with his vitals. They all indicated a normal condition. Only his heavily dilated pupils gave away signs of something being wrong. It was what we'd call today, "a bad trip". Then, when these signs abated, they were replaced by a strongly surreal feeling that made everything look like a first experience. The things that were familiar in Hofmann's world began to look new and he encountered them with a sense of genuine wonder.

Throughout the years from LSD's discovery, it has had its history retold by many and somewhere along the line, it was bestowed Christian and Eastern undertones. As we see though, that was never a part of its beginning. After the effects wore off, Hofmann was amazed. Not only was he somehow certain that LSD discovered him, he also envisaged its breakthrough strides in psychiatry. What he did not envisage was that it would become something people subject to misuse, taking it for pleasure and hurting themselves in the process. He would later observe however, that the phenomenon was a coping mechanism: young people seeking an escape from the cruel world in which they lived. He was sure that much of our unhappiness came from the fact that we were no longer in tune with nature; our sense of wonder had been eroded by technology and other modern-day dynamics that made us less human. He became an advocate of spiritual rejuvenation and a re-joining with elements of nature, and he said as much at that centennial celebration in 2006. To many, Hofmann was the creator of a religion which deviated from all others. In his religion, everyone could have the exact level of spiritual enlightenment experienced by the founder. But just as he was considered a force among mystics and their lot, he was also highly revered in science. This is phenomenal in the sense that those two worlds hardly ever collide, being usually skeptical and disapproving of each other. Researchers across different fields of medicine and pharmacy looked forward to investigating the effects and possibilities of LSD in curing stubborn mental diseases and improving human understanding of consciousness. Such scientists and researchers were known for their often-unfounded enthusiasm, but this time, it seemed there was really something to be excited about.

The second incident that indicated a new dawn for psychedelic drugs research was a court ruling. It was the year 2006 when the United States Supreme Court ruled in favor of a religious group- UDV- importing their psychedelic tea into the United States. Even though the Buh government was strongly against it at the time, the courts agreed, quoting the Religious Freedom Restoration Act of 1993. Not only did the ruling increase membership for the religious clique, it also stirred something in a lot of Americans; something that had to do with religious rejuvenation. The Supreme Court's decision meant that it was legal to use psychedelic drugs, as long as they were for religious purposes. It is yet to be seen if this was a right decision but it did herald a sort of departure from what had been obtainable regarding psychedelic drugs.

The third event was the publication of psychedelic research carried out by scientist Roland Griffiths. Surprisingly, Griffiths set out to examine the interaction between a psychedelic- Psilocybin- and mystical experiences, and as it turned out, he was doing it as a result of a mystical experience he had himself. Published in a journal called Psychopharmacology, the paper had the most widespread impact on the resurrection of psychedelic research. It was covered by the press and had comments from prominent drug researchers like Charles Schuster and Herbert D. Kleber. Much of the excitement surrounding this paper was from the possibility that Psilocybin- as well as other psychedelics- could be used in treating addiction and other mental illnesses. Also prominent in the paper was a fundamental clarification. For so long, psychedelics have been lumped together: the traditional psychedelics versus other abused drugs. The former include LSD, Psilocybin, Mescaline and DMT, and are in a completely different class from other drugs with their damaging and addictive effects.

Needless to say, Griffiths' paper deviates from what one would expect from a scientist. Instead of studying Psilocybin as a potential cure for mental illness, Griffiths examined its place in the realm of spirituality with humans who were hale and hearty. As one psychiatrist noted, maybe it was time for scientists to acknowledge the existence of experiences beyond the confines of science. If there ever was a typical man expected to be interested in psychedelics, Griffiths wasn't him. He was one of those men who came across as stiff. His clothes; his posture; his demeanor; all these exuded order and discipline.

Griffiths was raised in California where he attended Occidental college as a Psychology major. He went on to study Psychopharmacology at the University of Minnesota where he took up interest in studying behaviors that led to drug use and addictions. During his entire education, he never came across psychedelics as a viable field of research. Immediately after grad school, Griffiths began working with Johns Hopkins, where he has done a lot of phenomenal work in analyzing substances and patterns of dependence, addiction, and withdrawal. He was widely published, and by the time he clocked 50, he was an established name in the world of science; a renowned scientist at the top of his craft. Little did he know, that he was going to experience certain unforeseen events that would change a lot of who he had been all his life.

First, he was randomly introduced to Siddha Yoga. Interestingly, Griffiths had always shown interest in the understanding of consciousness. He had even tried out meditation while in school but that didn't work out. For some unexplainable reason however, when his friend introduced him to Siddha Yoga in 1994, he got it. His interest in meditation and the higher realm grew steadily, eventually overwhelming his interest in science. While he battled his inner scientist- who was of course not comfortable with all these new opposing knowledge- he also found it hard to relate within his usual circle anymore. He was surrounded by scientists who thought anything that was not scientifically proven was not worth a thought. But Griffiths found himself becoming more immersed with each passing day. He had a supernatural experience which he referred to as an awakening and only spoke vaguely of. The more he experienced this new dimensions through meditation, the more his thirst grew. He was going to quit science and move to India in pursuit of these new experiences when Charles Schuster came along.

Schuster's call to Griffiths proved life-changing indeed. The former head of the National Institute on Drug Abuse told his friend about Bob Jesse, a computer scientist who had made it his personal quest to resuscitate psychedelics. Jesse had recently held a meeting with religious intellectuals, research experts, and therapists to discuss the spiritual and curative possibilities of Psychedelics. Schuster taught Griffiths should listen to Jesse's ideas on working with entheogens.

Jesse would become one of two non-scientists whose efforts contributed in no small measure to the resuscitation of psychedelics. The other man was Rick Doblin, and like Jesse, he had witnessed first-hand the incredible mind-altering capabilities of psychedelics. They were convinced these drugs had a lot of good to offer the world, and spared no expense in finding scientific proof for their belief. Doblin is one of those people who just never give up. He had been on the trail as far back as 1986 when psychedelics were considered as nothing short of evil. He established the Multidisciplinary Association for Psychedelic Studies (MAPS) during that time. Doblin had used LSD and MDMA while in college and became somehow convinced that he was meant to be a psychedelic therapist. But after the ban on MDMA, that dream was threatened. In his quest to influence federal laws in favor of psychedelics, he enrolled at Harvard's Kennedy School for a doctorate in public policy. He was that determined. His final paper laid the groundwork for so much of the progress that Psilocybin and MDMA are making today. His approach is sometimes seen as disorganized but this is largely due to his personality. Doblin is what you might call a free-spirit. He openly speaks to the press about his psychedelic encounters and chosen strategy in his quest. He does not hide the fervor with which he pursues federal approval for psychedelics, and his home and office are testament to that as well. He openly shares how he not just wants approval for the drugs, but also wants their integration into the society. He ruffles feathers- sometimes with more precautious fellow soldiers like Bob Jesse- but has never slowed down. Despite all these, Doblin has been able to fund studies establishing the potential of MDMA in treating Post-Traumatic Stress Disorder (PTSD). He believes strongly that psychedelics are not only beneficial for therapeutic reasons but that they can unite the human race by revealing a shared supernatural form of consciousness irrespective of our perceived differences.

Bob Jesse, on the other hand, is a completely different man. Probably the only thing he has in common with Doblin is their work with psychedelics. There's nothing haphazard about this man. He avoids the press and even when he speaks, his words are always carefully selected, which is why he's a man of few words. He lives all by himself in a not-so-modern cabin on a mountaintop and is far from all forms of modernization, save for his internet. His cabin was too little to fit two people so my visit with him was held outside, among the trees. Not surprisingly, he declined having his picture taken for any reason. Yes, this man is out in the woods, but speaking with him makes you realize that he has a comprehensive strategy- a grand design involving Griffiths. Upon closer interaction, you discover that this man packs a lot within his willowy frame.

Jesse studied computer science and electrical engineering at Johns Hopkins and worked at Bell Labs in his twenties. It was at Bell that his 'puppet master' persona would develop. When he came out as gay, he convinced the management to take a couple of actions in support of the gay and lesbian community. He derived ultimate pleasure from knowing he achieved milestones, and demanded no recognition. He repeated the feat when he moved to Oracle in 1990. His first awareness of psychedelics was in high school when he listened to a drug education talk. Of all the classes discussed that day, he was intrigued by the psychedelics. He liked the fact that it was not addictive and when the teacher spoke about accompanying visual perceptions, he was hooked and yearning to know more. But he would not quench that thirst until much later, precisely, while working at Bell Labs.

He and a group of friends would experiment with psychedelics every Saturday afternoon. During all of their sessions, they made sure there was always one person who was not as 'high' as the rest. Each Saturday afternoon also saw an increase in the previous one's dosage. He had no idea what lay ahead of him the particular Saturday afternoon.

He had taken in a large dosage of LSD as usual but he wasn't prepared for the encounter he witnessed next. It was so out-of-this-world that he struggles to describe it in words. After losing all consciousness of his physical space- the room he was in and the friends that surrounded him- he floated into a new dimension of consciousness where he was a floating observer in something like a supernatural depiction of a creation story. He confesses that he was awed about the experience but there was nothing scary about it. That singular experience converted a science believer into someone who believed in more. He no longer believed that the brain was the seat of all consciousness. He believed there was more out there.

Personally, I wondered what made these encounters any different from dreams and nightmares. We all have them, but they do not usually leave us with a strong sense of conviction that fuels causes such as the one championed by Jesse and

Doblin. Same with drug-induced illusions. People don't hold on to them as strongly as these psychedelic encounters. So what gives? For one, it's likely that these experiences possess noetic quality- the feeling that one has been let in on a life-altering secret. Such convictions are hard to shake off. Science, however, does not believe in such theories. People like James and Doblin claim to have gone beyond the waking consciousness to experience something the human senses cannot, but it is all in the head. There is no scientific way of establishing its truthfulness.

Supernatural encounters usually make it difficult- near impossible- for people to differentiate between the inside and the outside, and subsequently, what is true and what is not. Bob Jesse's experience was so phenomenal that he began to explore other means of religious expression like meditation and Buddhism. Before long, he was considering making this pursuit his life's work. Being a computer engineer was not so fulfilling anymore. He founded the Council on Spiritual Practices (CSP) through which he promoted psychedelics- which he called entheogens.

After moving to San Francisco, he wasted no time getting in touch with prominent names in the psychedelic field. There was James Fadiman, the psychologist who initiated research into psychedelics and problem solving. There was Myron Stolaroff, Fadiman's colleague who, after an acid trip, abandoned engineering for research on psychedelics. There was Sasha and Ann Shulgin, prominent Psychedelic enthusiasts. Finally, there was Huston Smith, religion scholar who had once been in a psychedelic experiment. All these were folks who had been on the path long before Jesse and he was determined to get a lot from them.

Combined with his extensive reading, he uncovered a lot that had been buried concerning psychedelics. He discovered that, from the 1950s to the 1970s, there had been studies and experiments which recorded remarkable results in using psychedelics to treat several conditions. He also realized that many of those studies and experiments suffered the problem of bias, not measuring up to cotemporary scientific standards. But in the end, Jesse was more intrigued by studies indicating psychedelics were found to benefit healthy humans, that is, it also enhanced people who are not sick. One of such studies was the 1962 Good Friday experiment carried out by Walter Pahnke, Timothy Leary's PhD student who also happened to be psychiatrist and a minister. In the experiment, divinity students who were given Psilocybin mentioned having had spiritual encounters that drew them closer to God. It was in the same experiment that Doblin and

Jesse would later find inconsistencies respectively. Researcher bias was established as it was later found out that Pahnke did not record everything that went on during the experiment. He conveniently left out the part of one of his subjects experiencing temporary insanity.

Jesse and Doblin were interested in the results of such studies, but if they were to present them as evidence in their cause, the experiment would have to be recreated in compliance to standard scientific procedure. Jesse had the journals and books to bring him up to speed on the subject he was so passionate about. He also had several people who were authorities on the matter. Then there was the Esalen Institute, retreat center of sorts. Since its establishment in 1962, Esalen has been the go-to place for healing and spiritual enthusiasts. It was where Czech immigrant psychiatrist Stanislav Grof, did a lot of his work. Grof is one of the foremost proponents of using LSD as a therapeutic tool in psychotherapy. Till this day, most of the therapists still using psychedelics in their practice, are students of Grof. After LSD was banned however, the teachings on psychedelics stopped at Esalen. However, enthusiasts of psychedelics still use the place as venue for their meetings and discussions, and by the first month in 1994, Jesse had succeeded in getting an invite to one of such. The year was starting to look up for the psychedelic proponents.

There was a new administrator at the FDA who was giving psychedelics a fair fighting chance. Psychiatrist, Rick Strassman and the duo of Rick Doblin and Charles Grob were conducting approved trials on DMT and MDMA respectively. So there was a lot of hope going around, and for these enthusiasts who had mostly lived in the shadows, even the slightest ray of hope was something. They needed to organize and concentrate all their efforts to make the most of the opportunities opening up. They set the meeting for Esalen, and when Jesse heard of it at the Shulgins' he asked to attend.

When, during the meeting, he realized how little they were focused on the spiritual benefits of psychedelics, he knew he had to do something. In less than two years, CSP was established and hosting its own meeting at Esalen. For the most part, Jesse invited authorities in Psychedelics research, therapists, and spiritual leaders. But he also extended an invite to an unusual person, Schuster. For some unexplainable reason, he just thought a man with whom he had no prior relationship might want to come to such a meeting. I would later find out from Schuster's widow that he was an open-minded man, but Jesse did not know this at the time. As it turned out, Schuster attended the meeting and actually enjoyed being there. He also made notable contributions to their discussion. He sounded a note of caution, advising Jesse against doing research on MDMA and LSD. Unlike Psilocybin, both drugs already had a bad reputation and too much political and cultural baggage. Later on, Schuster introduced Jesse to Griffiths and the two would eventually collaborate to produce the 2006 landmark study on psilocybin and mystic encounters.

Before the study took off, Griffiths noted that they needed a therapist on the team. Coincidentally, Jesse knew a psychologist, Bill Richards, whom he'd met some years back at a psychedelic gathering. Bill Richards could not have been a more fitting choice. Apart from Stan Grof, he was the one person who had the most experience with psychedelic inquiries. He had resorted to conventional psychotherapy after the drugs were banned but he never lost his interest in them. Richards was elated to join the team.

Richards had gone on his first 'trip' when he volunteered at the University of Göttingen's Department of Psychiatry. He was studying divinity in Yale but was at the time in Germany for a semester abroad. His first trip thrust him into a mystical consciousness that he found soothing and peaceful. Subsequent ones were however not so good. It wasn't until later while showing his friend, Walter Pahnke, how to go on a trip, that he had another good one. Pahnke had suggested Richards try it again in better room conditions and with a higher dosage. And it worked. Richards concluded 3 things from his mystical encounters:

1. Psychedelic trips are the same experience as the hallowed encounters narrated by mystics and they are both real.
2. Regardless of the cause- drugs or otherwise- mystical consciousness is the primeval foundation of religion.
3. Consciousness is not located in the brain. It is out there, in the cosmos. Our brains just pick up the signals.

Richards went on to work at Spring Grove state hospital in Baltimore. Contrary to what popular history tells us, Timothy Leary was not the only one conducting studies in psychedelics. In fact, Spring Grove conducted studies on which many other studies eventually built. They ran a program that saw many mental illness patients get treated with psychedelics, and were for so long the toast of the public with all their work. Even after it was widely believed that all studies and programs on psychedelics had been stopped, the Spring Grove LSD program was still very active. Not until money ran out did the program end. By that time, psychedelics- such as LSD- had become a societal ill and a subject of embarrassment among scientists.

The government's harsh reaction to psychedelics, according to many researchers, might not have been the case were it not for the actions of Timothy Leary. His loud advocacy occasioned the boom and subsequent misuse of these drugs, resulting in societal outcry and government clampdown. This, and a scandal involving the CIA made a shutdown of the Spring Grove program inevitable. Griffiths notes how incredible it is that such a promising scientific inquiry was shut down for reasons totally devoid of science.

When Griffiths, Jesse and Richards were about to commence with a pilot study in 1998, they met with a lot of discouraging remarks. But they pressed on, and after 5 stages of review, eventually got approval. Richards notes that during the first session of their study, he was overwhelmed all over again as he watched one of their volunteers obviously transcending dimensions.

Finally, in 1999, after 22 long years, Richards supervised the administration of a legal dose of psilocybin to an American.

Many more have followed since then, with varying groups such as cancer patients, and healthy people who just wanted to explore the mystical consciousness. My utmost interest was in the healthy normal. I was curious to know how this felt for them because theirs was a new aspect of this subject that was under investigation. But my curiosity was also piqued because I saw this group as the one I could most relate to; maybe knowing how it felt for them would give me an insight into how it would feel for me. But then again, I realized they were not like me in a very significant way. All of them were believers one way or the other; people with already-formed spiritual orientations. The program was more interested in studying spiritual effects so that was reflected in their choice of volunteers.

The team spared no effort in ensuring that this program was conducted in line with standard procedure. After many years of the experiment, many of the volunteers are still able to explain in detail what they experienced. For many, it started out scary of course, but because they had been assured before the trips, they eventually relaxed. There were accounts of floating in space, becoming one with the universe, meeting with a dead loved one, being healed, waking up with a transformed mind, etc. Comparing the accounts to Williams James' description of a mystical encounter, I was able to draw a line of correlation.

One of the volunteers recounts getting a profound insight, one he knows with a certainty (noetic quality) but finds almost embarrassing to admit: Love conquers all. As much as fifteen years later, these volunteers can still vividly recall their mystical experiences and how it translated in their normal lives. For most, there is a total mind transformation that has made it possible for them to pursue the lives they are really happy with.

But beyond the volunteers, guides who sit in while the volunteers go through their journeys have shared how their minds have been transformed by just watching others in their experience. As slightly envious as I was of these volunteers, I struggled with more questions. I wondered how one was to explain or measure these experiences. For instance, where do the kaleidoscopic patterns and images come from? Griffiths himself does not have an answer, but he does not disregard his volunteer's experiences anyway. He keeps an open mind, even at the risk of being ridiculed by many of his colleagues. His stand bears similarities to Williams James' conclusions about mystical states.

When Griffiths' friend introduced him to Siddha Yoga, he soon became disoriented with science and was well on his way out. After his work with Psilocybin however, his illuminated mind has rediscovered an interest in science. Unlike before however, he now does his work with an awareness of dimensions that science just cannot penetrate. Apart from the fact that he's been recognized with an award, their work has paved the way for an unprecedented number of studies into psychedelics.

Griffiths' new outlook involves an appreciation for the scientific as well as the non-scientific. He refuses to keep a closed mind concerning anything, and has no time to spare for those who do. He firmly believes that both dimensions can make up for each other's lapses and ultimately provide balanced answers to our biggest questions about life.

CHAPTER 2: NATURAL HISTORY Bemushroomed

Key Notes:

- *Mushrooms are the primary source of psilocybin*
- *It is not exactly clear why mushrooms produce such a strong chemical in their fruit.*
- *The location of psilocybin in mushrooms strikes out the defense mechanism explanation*
- *Paul Stamets believed in what he called a network of nature. He believed psilocybin is an Earth messenger sent to humans.*
- *Fungi- one of the most overlooked groups- are essential to our planet's survival*
- *Psilocybin mushrooms were originally used by the Natives for healing and divination*

When I took my first meeting with Griffiths, I did not expect to leave at the end with a gift. And if I had thought of a gift, it would not have been what he handed to me after I answered a pre-gift question. He asked me if I was aware that I was aware at that very moment and I said yes. The gift was a coin. Engraved on one side was the psilocybin mushroom, and on the other, a William Blake Quote. He had a lot of that coin which he gave to every volunteer on their way out. I doubt many of them knew that the substance they had just taken in came from the mushroom, sometimes called magic mushroom.

Discovered by science in the 1950s, the Mazatec Indians in southern Mexico had been using it for therapeutic and spiritual, purposes. They called it the flesh of the gods. But this interesting piece of history is hardly remembered today. Thanks to Albert Hofmann, the psilocybin used today is synthesized and available in capsules that look and taste nothing like the mushrooms. It's easy to sum it all up to modernity in science, but there is more here. There are efforts to dissociate psilocybin from its origins and nature that are reminiscent of divination by Native Americans.

After spending some days around the Hopkins Laboratory, my interest in these natural sources was piqued. I was curious to know why and how the mushrooms produced their psychoactive substance. The easiest explanation would be that it was a defense mechanism, but the fact that they produced it in their fruit strikes that explanation out. The fruit is that part of their body they want predators to eat so why would psilocybin be concentrated there? On another level, one can decide to query the philosophical issues therein. It stands to logic that since these experiences are brought on by the presence of a chemical, we wouldn't be wrong to conclude that whatever mystical consciousness is experienced is only a misunderstood chemical reaction, right? Yet, people who have had such encounters are very convinced that it is not the case; that it is something beyond what we know as reality. What, to me, was an easily deduced case of chemical reaction, was to them a supernatural encounter confirming that there truly is something else 'out there'.

I set out on an inquiry into the little brown mushrooms- or LBMs as they're mostly called- and hoped it would shed some light on the situation. I needed someone who was familiar with these mushrooms; who could keep me from getting myself killed by poisoning. That person was Paul Stamets. Not only had Stamets studied mushrooms all his life, he had published extensive information on the *Psilocybe* category of mushrooms. So, yes, he was an authority, but he was also a peculiar man. He did not identify with the academy or have a graduate degree, but you'd be wrong to imagine him thinking less of himself for those reasons. In fact, he can brag to a fault. He provides funding for his research and never hesitates to boast about how much mushroom knowledge he has. It becomes more interesting when he tells you how he comes about the knowledge:

information shared with him by the mushrooms in question. You can also often hear him talking about his work with the Pentagon's Defense Advanced Research Projects Agency (DARPA) and the National Institutes of Health (NIH).

Born in Salem, Ohio, Stamets' passion lies in a subject that is mostly disregarded. Even though our world as we know it cannot survive without fungi, we continue to treat them like outcasts. Stamets is very adamant about his assertions that mushrooms are the answer to a lot of the world's problems-pollution, cancer, bioterrorism, insect infestation, you name it! In a nutshell, Paul Stamets is consumed by mushrooms. But not only was Stamets more occupied than when I had seen him last, he had also recently being recognized by two American science societies. For a man who had never been on the same page with scientific explanations, that was a big deal. I feared that Stamets was no longer a free agent; that he'd be unable to be my guide on my mushroom trail.

Fortunately, that was not the case. He was happy, in fact to help me and he mentioned that he was in the process of updating his publication of psilocybes. He told me where I could find the Psilocybe azurescens and when I could find them with fruit. The time was after thanksgiving and I couldn't wait. To keep myself occupied, I read Stamets' guide on Psilocybes. Over two hundred species of psilocybes are scattered worldwide, popping up on distressed land. The distress could be caused by ecological disaster- such as floods and storms- or deliberate disaster- such as bulldozing. They survive on dead plants and manure. Interestingly, it appears mushrooms have a preference for the distressed lands of our own doing so they're found more in the cities than in the forest. One would imagine then, that finding little brown mushrooms would be pretty easy. Wrong. In fact, the more I perused Stamets' guide, the more confused I got. There was not just a ton of mushrooms, there were a ton of mushroom features as well, and it wasn't easy keeping up with them long enough to find what I was looking for. It didn't exactly help that I came across a chapter on mistaken identity of mushrooms. Stamets clearly warned against going mushroom picking without adequate knowledge. It could mean the difference between life and death. I even attempted identifying psilocybin mushrooms with something he calls 'The Stametsian Rule'. In the end however, I chose to wait for my meeting with the mushroom expert himself. My stay at Stamets' was enlightening and exhausting.

Not surprisingly, he lived in a huge house surrounded by trees and before I could settle in, provided me with the story of how mushrooms built the house. At first, the flow of new information and speculation I was getting was refreshing, but soon enough it became a torrent, and I grew legitimately tired of hearing how everything in the world always comes back to fungi. Stamets is one of those people you come across and wonder *how did he get here?*

From a young age, Stamets had developed deep-seated admiration for his older brother, John. John was five years his senior but Stamets looked up to him like he was more than human. The fact that the older boy kept a laboratory in their basement made him very cool to his younger brother who equated the laboratory to heaven. When John was fifteen, he told 14-year old Paul Stamets about magic mushrooms, but before he could explain any further, went away to Yale. Among some of the things he did not pack to Yale was a book titled *"Altered states of consciousness"*.

The book had such a huge effect on Stamets, and not because it was a compilation of extraordinary mental states but because of the extreme responses it seemed to provoke in some people. A friend of Stamets once borrowed it from him and his parents burned it. Their actions strengthened Stamets' resolve to know by all means what information this book carried that folks were so scared of. While in college,

Stamets, who was so good with mushrooms because he was always looking down, trying to avoid talking to people because of his stuttering, had a psychedelic experience. He had mistakenly eaten an overdose of psilocybin mushrooms. Stamets left that experience with a transformed mind, singularity of purpose, and no more stuttering. So driven was he that in no time, he had become an authority on the psilocybe genus.

He dropped out of Kenyon College and joined another college that was only in an experimental phase. He teamed up with like minds Michael Beug, Jeremy Bigwood and Jonathan Ott to study extensively, the psilocybin mushrooms. They were doing this at a time when psilocybin was illegal and its study, avoided by researchers. Already, it was being classified by some as a LSD-alternative. Stamets and his colleagues made news in no time. They were doing phenomenal work with psilocybins, and most significantly, taking the psilocybe spotlight away from southern Mexico to the Pacific Northwest. They were soon considered as leading authorities on the subject and regularly held conferences where psychedelics could come together and deliberate. Thanks to psilocybin-spiked drinks, these conferences turned out to be more of wild parties than official symposiums. Still, it afforded Stamets some of the greatest opportunities of his lifetime. He got to meet R. Gordon Wasson, the first man to discover and experience Psilocybin outside the Native Indians of southern Mexico. His piece in Life magazine is considered today as what initiated the psychedelic movement in the US. Stamets later gave me one of the original copies of that historical 1957 magazine issue. He had been collecting them over the years.

As it happened, Wasson was a newly-married man in the year 1927. He and his Russian bride, during one of their leisurely strolls, would come upon a path of mushrooms. His wife suggested making dinner with those mushrooms but Wasson would have none of it. Wasson and his wife, a physician, were interested in finding out what influenced both opposite reactions they had towards the mushrooms. Their working theory was that our forebears had worshipped a mushroom ages ago. They then set out to find that divine mushroom that drew people closer to God.

After an intensive search during which Wasson focused more on Asia, he would find out that what he was traveling the world for was right there in Mexico and Central America. He would later find these groups where the locals held the psilocybin mushroom in high regard. To them, it was sacred and they guarded its secret jealously. They had cause to. The

Spanish had earlier engaged in a series of activities designed to suppress the mushrooms. The attacks were rooted in a fundamental fear that the mushrooms would render irrelevant and powerless, the institution called the church.

It wasn't until 1955, on a night in June, that Wasson would eat his first mushrooms. His observation notes record the same experiences had by those who take the drug. Wasson was sure his theory had been proven right after he returned from the mystical experience. Timothy Leary, along with probably the whole of America, would read Wasson's article. There were also TV appearances where he shared his experiences, and soon, he was administering to other interested folks, the mushrooms he had brought back with him.

Wasson sent some of the mushrooms to Hofmann who upon eating them, confirmed that they worked just like the synthesized pills. Wasson then gave the pills to the local healer who had introduced him to the mushroom in Huautla. She also confirmed that the pills acted exactly as the mushrooms. Sadly, the quiet town would come to be besieged by a frantic demand for the mushrooms. Sabina, the local healer would face condemnation for giving away the people's well-guarded secret and bringing foreigners to invade their sacred space. Wasson blamed himself for what befell Sabina and her town as a result of his actions.

Terence McKenna with his stoned ape theory was another mushroom believer who was driving an interesting conversation. McKenna suggested that the consumption of psilocybin mushrooms by our evolutionary ancestors, the apes, in some way triggered evolution into Homo sapiens. While at Stamets', I wondered again what it was about these mushrooms that gave people experiences from which they emerged with new convictions; convictions that they stood strongly by and were eager to share it with the world. Imagine seeing this from the mushroom's eye. The Homo sapiens are a resourceful specie. Having their interest and enthusiasm would serve their own interests too!

Stamets and I would eventually set out for our mushroom-gathering expedition. After setting up camp in one of the parks bordering the Columbia River, we stepped out. It was a long walk, and Stamets made sure to keep it going with his mycological chatter. There were a couple of LBMs along the way, but after an hour, we still had not come across one with psilocybin. Some two hours later however, Stamets found one, and we went on to find seven in total that day. After finding the first one, I bruised the stipe at Stamets' instruction, and sure enough, a blue tinge appeared, indicating the presence of psilocin. By the next day, I was catching on enough to pick out a few psilocybin mushrooms of my own. After drying our collection, I was eager to try one already. When Stamets, the mushroom expert, told me that Psilocybe azurescens- *or azzies*- have been known to temporary paralyze the eater, my enthusiasm abated. Maybe not now.

Throughout that weekend, I struggled with the question of why the mushroom would produce a chemical that profoundly affects the minds of animals that feed on it. What did the mushroom stand to gain? Italian ethnobotanist, Giorgio Samorini, posits in his book that when members of a species are faced with sudden and unfamiliar crisis- environmentally or otherwise- it is sometimes best for embers to forgo their conditioned response patterns and try new behaviors. That got me thinking. Are we at that point of crisis where we need to depart from familiar and conditioned patterns? Maybe nature is trying to tell us something by bringing psychedelic substances our way.

This was the type of theory Stamets would have no trouble subscribing to. During our camping, he would tell me how psilocybin was sent by the earth to deliver us a message and we were to take heed if we wanted to avoid destruction. Humans, according to him, had been chosen for this message because of our sophisticated language and capacity for consciousness. Much of Stamets' talk actually were similar to the accounts I recorded from the volunteers in Griffiths' Hopkins Lab. He spoke like one who had transcended the waking consciousness and was on a mission to get everyone to accept whatever convictions he had gotten from that experience. I found most of his words incredulous and was almost tuning off when I remembered the tour of Fungi Perfecti that this peculiar man had given me. He had set up the company right out of college, brimming with passion s usual. I thought of all the research rooms and laboratories I visited there; all the work that had been done and those that were still being done. I realized that even if Stamets did tend to go a little extra on the talk, at least he was walking the walk. I had no idea what category to place him in but I was convinced that this man was a scientist.

Several weeks later, after coming across a biography on Alexandra von Humboldt, the great early nineteenth-century German scientist, I would see how much he sounded and acted like Stamets. They were romantic scientists, respecting and interacting with nature in all its forms, unlike modern scientists who disregard nature's dynamics, choosing to isolate and objectify it in a laboratory.

Months later, my wife, Judith and I, crumbled the mushrooms I had picked with Stamets and made a glass of tea out of it. The effects kicked in first with Judith and it did not look much like a calming experience. She preferred to lie on the couch in the dark. I took some more of my mushroom tea because I wasn't feeling anything yet. Then, I stepped out towards the garden. This was where my experience started to kick in, and what an experience it was! Interestingly, I had a lot of interaction with the plants and leaves and trees. I saw them alive than I had ever seen them before. They glowed with a kind of brilliance I had never seen before and I could see them watching me. The garden at the back of the house came alive and I could feel myself flowing in tandem with the dragonflies and the flowers and the trees. I had been in that garden countless times but this was the first time I was really *being* there.

At the end of the day, I wasn't quite sure what to make of my experiences. I felt like I had a mystical encounter of sorts, and I felt my heart opening up anew. I could chalk it up to my earlier suggestion of it being a mere chemical reaction, or I could attribute it to something beyond me, out there.

However, I was surprised that my experiences that day did not require any mystical understanding. Sure, there was an intense consciousness not similar to the normal reality, but I did not need mystical powers to interpret them. Prior to my experience, I was so sure that entrance into the realm of divinity did not require a belief in the spiritual. But after the azzies, I was not so sure anymore. I was no longer absolute. Now, I was open and ready to re-analyze my explanations.

CHAPTER 3: HISTORY The First Wave

Key Notes:

- *Contrary to popular opinion, Timothy Leary did not pioneer psychedelic research*

- *Leary shared similar beliefs with most psychedelic researchers. He was just the only one vocal and arrogant enough to say it anywhere*

- *Psychedelics were first considered as psychosis-inducing drugs*

- *Huxley's book "Doors of Perception" shaped popular perception of psychedelic experiences.*

- *The actions of Leary led to the banning of psychedelics in 1966. He blurred whatever lines there were between their healing potential and mystical experiences*

- *Instead of shutting down as widely thought, most psychedelic researchers only took their work underground*

It is no coincidence that Timothy Leary seems to be written all over the history of psychedelics, making it seem like psychedelic research began with his 1960 Harvard Psilocybin study and ended when he was shut down in 1963 by political and cultural opposition. Basic research into that history might make this seem like the case, but it is not so. Leary achieved that status after acting on advice from media guru, Marshall McLuhan. The latter gave him some tips on how to position himself in the press, and sure enough, it worked. Yet, anyone who bothers to go beyond mainstream information will uncover facts detailing extensive research programs that had been going on in various places long before Leary must have discovered psychedelics. California, Vancouver, England; these were only some of the places where researchers, scientists, therapists, and other enthusiasts had been studying psychedelics, testing hypotheses and formulating theories on which future uses of the drugs would be based.

Then Leary came much later with his style of advocacy, ruffling the feathers of government and the society. His approach led to the banning of psychedelics and any inquiries into it, putting an end to the hard work of all his predecessors. There are other researchers- like Stephen Ross- who came to discover the real history of psychedelics. Ross' moment came when a colleague told him that LSD had once been used to treat numerous alcoholics in the U.S and Canada. He dug deeper into research and was stunned to find all the phenomenal works that were not related to Leary. He was specializing in the treatment of addiction, so much of what he uncovered was very useful. What he had been told- or more appropriately, not being told since psychedelics became a sort of taboo in science- was very different from what he was finding out.

In 1950, LSD's entrance into the world of psychiatry brought along with it a barrage of questions regarding its use and application. Scientists and therapists were working hard at understanding the drug, but the CIA was doing something similar, in secret of course. They were trying to figure out the possibilities inherent in LSD- mind control instrument, truth serum, or chemical defense.

After Hofmann's 1943 LSD trip, Sandoz, the company for which he worked embarked on a mission to find out what exactly they had on their hands. They sent out free samples of the drug to any researcher or therapist who indicated interest and could analyze the drug to see what it could be used for. To a large extent, this was accountable for the initial boom of psychedelic research, and when the controversy that trailed it got to a head in 1966, Sandoz withdrew the drug. Before the withdrawal however, a lot had been discovered about this new drug and psychedelics in general. For one, psychedelic experiences were found to be highly influenced by prior expectations of the individual.

There was also the Aldous Huxley twist. The renowned writer and Eastern mysticism proponent was given mescaline by a scientist who needed Huxley's words to accurately describe the psychedelic experience. Huxley recorded his experience in the 1954 book *Doors of Perception*. Not surprisingly, his account was tinged heavily with eastern mysticism and that perception has come to be regarded as part of psychedelic drugs today, influencing the descriptions of many others who went through the experience. But is Huxley's book a true depiction of the psychedelic experience or an account of his own expectation-tinged experience? During that time also, researchers who tested psychedelic drugs on themselves showed a remarkable change in disposition towards the research than their counterparts who did not. They displayed unfounded enthusiasm that many thought would bias the results of their work. Finally, there was the challenge of fitting psychedelics into the standard construction of science. So many of its elements demanded subjectivity that could not be accommodated in modern science.

The journey to the name "psychedelics" was a long one. The names changed as new findings were made on the compositions, actions and effects of these drugs. LSD was initially called a Psychotomimetic because those who took it- and later Psilocybin- displayed symptoms of psychosis patients. This contributed to the first widespread suggestion of LSD. It was thought that the drug may actually not have curative powers, but it could help further the understanding of psychosis.

One man whose role in this field is often ignored is Humphry Osmond. Osmond was a psychiatrist at St. George's Hospital in London who worked with schizophrenic patients. When a friend told him about mescaline causing hallucinations similar to schizophrenic hallucinations, he was interested in knowing more. Both men, also researchers, began to consider studying whether schizophrenia was triggered by a chemical imbalance in the body. Osmond however did not get the support he needed from St. George so he began looking elsewhere. That elsewhere turned out to be Canada, at the Saskatchewan Mental Hospital in Weyburn. In no time, the hospital became the nucleus of psychotomimetics research.

For the most part, their research positioned psychedelics as drugs that produced horrific bouts of insanity, until one day when Osmond and his Canadian colleague, Abram Hoffer, casually noted how the psychedelic experience was similar to the delirium tremens which usually preceded an alcoholic's conviction to remain sober. That heralded the beginning of a series of research that aimed to establish the effectiveness of psychedelics in curing alcoholic addiction. Half of the subjects used in the research were cured of their addiction, opening up a new approach to studying psychedelics: considering the experience and not the chemical.

Although this new approach was phenomenal and widely embraced by therapists, the results were largely different from what was in existence. Instead of insanity bouts, volunteers were now describing feelings of peace and oneness with the world. This forced Osmond and his team to look into their model again. They came to realize that it was possible they were calling insanity what was actually transcendence. They also had not taken into consideration the set and setting in which the drugs were administered, and as it turned out, this was an important element. Nevertheless, LSD eventually acquired a wonder-drug status for treating alcohol addiction, and even though it had a lot of critics, it was policy-backed as standard treatment option for alcohol addiction.

Bill Wilson was the co-founder of Alcoholics Anonymous, and in the mid-1950s, he was interested in LSD. He wasn't so perplexed by the idea because a similar experience had helped him overcome his own addiction in 1934. He would later take part in sever LSD sessions with Sidney Cohen and Betty Eisner. Cohen was a specialist in internal medicine at the Brentwood VA hospital. Wilson had met him through Humphry Osmond. Eisner was a young psychologist who, not too long ago, had completed her doctorate at UCLA. Wilson took two things away from his experiences during these sessions:

1. LSD trips were nothing like the delirium tremens experienced by alcoholics
2. Nevertheless, the LSD experience could spark the kind of divine awakening that led to sobriety.

The latter suggested that Alcoholics Anonymous could benefit from the use of LSD in treating addiction. Wilson was on board with this idea but the other members of management kicked against it.

Cohen and his colleagues were instrumental to the topping of the psychotomimetic concept. Because the psychosis that was a major part of the first research findings turned out to be inconsistent, and because there were new contradictory insights into the drug, researchers knew there was need for an improvement. Ronald Sandison, an English psychiatrist, coined the concept "Psycholytic", meaning "mind loosening". For some time, this was widely accepted. Cohen and his colleagues used LSD in treating their therapy patients and the rate of success was incredibly high. Stan Grof also found that using LSD moderately on his patients freed their minds so much that some were able to remember their births. Under the psycholytic paradigm, LSD became increasingly popular. The press was rife with reports of Hollywood celebrities who were testifying to the transforming effects of LSD, and as it usually happens in such cases, the high demand included those who were interested in using it indiscriminately. Reports of LSD being sold on the streets and therapists holding LSD parties under the disguise of therapy sessions were everywhere. Not too long after these, cultural undertones began to accompany the mention of LSD. Cohen grew increasingly uncomfortable at the events that were unfolding. He did not like the fact that LSD was considered more as having mystical qualities than scientific capabilities. The differences in experiences as narrated by those who use it also bore the tell-tale signs of expectancy effect. Cohen would continue to express his confidence in the therapeutic quality of LSD. He was particularly vocal about its success rate in curing anxiety in cancer patients. But he was never one to completely veer off the paths of science and he would constantly scold his colleagues whose irrational enthusiasm about the drug placed them on a path exactly opposite science.

Eventually, it was Osmond and Hoffer who would come up with the name that sticks till this day- Psychedelics. When the psychotomimetic theory collapsed, both men went to work on a new medicinal model to capture the new discoveries. With the help of two unlikely men- Aldous Huxley and Al Hubbard- they came up with the new model which provided a definite number of drugs to be included within its classification. Osmond and Hoffer insist that the features of the psychedelic therapy design were thought of by Al Hubbard, an unlikely science- or any other field for that matter- hero. Hubbard had at various times in his life been a spy, ex-con, gunrunner, inventor, and catholic mystic, among other things. Yet, it was Hubbard who set in motion the event that would later culminate in the prominence of psychedelics in Cultural Revolution, and to a large extent, his activities also led to the popularity of LSD in what is today known as the Silicon Valley.

No doubt, Timothy Leary's actions are largely to blame for the fate that eventually befell the field of psychedelics, but even without his loudness, LSD would have gotten them there on its own. Once it found its way to the streets, the attendant abuse unleashed consequences that were terrifying.

Although Leary had a reputation already by the time he resumed at Harvard, most did not know that he was becoming disillusioned with his line of work. He once conducted an experiment that showed psychotherapy had no real effect on the wellbeing of a patient. He was at that point where he was questioning his career. Leary became quite popular early on in Harvard, and not entirely for the right reasons: he was a rebel against institution, he had a history of misconduct with female students, and regularly spoke disdainfully of psychological inquiry. So even before his infamous Psilocybin project, he already had a reputation, and by the time he would have his psilocybin experience in 1960, he came back with a strong conviction to share the great knowledge he had received.

Leary enlisted the help of assistant professor, Richard Alpert on the Harvard Psilocybin Project, and together they carried out numerous psilocybin sessions. Although most of Leary's papers suggest that he was covering entirely new territory, the only new significant contribution he made to the field of study was the conceptualization of "set" and "setting". Leary was also popular for his outrageous research findings found to be filled with inconsistencies. Eventually, it became clear that this man of science was no longer interested in science; his interest in psilocybin was spiritually inclined. The institution of Harvard kicked against it but the rebellious Leary was not one to back down. After a while, the controversy made it to the press, hastening the outright banning of psychedelics research, the excommunication of Leary from Harvard, and his subsequent assumption of a spiritual personality.

Leary was adamant. He went on to establish the International Federation for Internal Freedom, a machinery for his continued propagation of the gospel of psychedelics in culture. By this time, every psychedelics researcher to have gone before and come after Leary were against him. His flagrant arrogance was putting all their work in jeopardy, as there were talks already of the government's frustration with him. The society was also now beginning to turn against every psychedelic drug, now that Leary was completely disregarding the therapeutic properties and promoting the mystical experience narrative.

Leary would go on to face nationwide embarrassment, living out much of his life on the run, in courts, jails, solitary confinement, and exile. He also wrote a couple of memoirs and appeared on TV shows. In all, he never seemed to lose his enthusiasm for the psychedelics in popular culture. Alpert went on to embark on a spiritual journey to India, returning as Ram Dass.

Although Leary was vocal and brazen, he was not the only one who was working towards incorporating psychedelics into the American culture. Novelist, Ken Kesey, had unknowingly signed up for a CIA-initiated program created to test the possibilities of using LSD as a weapon. When Kesey realized he had been used as a guinea-pig, he embarked on a mission to introduce the drugs to every young American.

The public outcry that followed was deafening, and of course, the press was not left out. The prevailing narrative now was a constant demonization of psychedelics. It did not help that the 1960s saw a rise in the number of young people who were experiencing anxiety, panic attacks, and even psychosis as a result of using psychedelics. Psychedelics, by the very nature of the experiences they brought, were a threat to the establishment and institution culture in which society had been ordered for so long. Leary was a threat because he encouraged young people to embrace experiences that turned them against the usually unnatural dictates of such establishments. Now however, Leary's greatest achievement appears to be the awakening of a generation that today, are at the helm of affairs in those institutions. Perhaps the atmosphere is now most conducive for a resuscitation of psychedelic research.

Psychedelic research and the drugs themselves were eventually banned in 1966, but as it turned out, most of the research only went underground, maintaining radio silence.

CHAPTER 4: TRAVELOGUE
Journeying Underground

Key Notes:

- *Underground psychedelic practice turned out to be as structured as the unhindered fields of science*
- *Ultimately, true freedom comes with a departure of one's ego*

Going on my own psychedelic journey did not look like it was going to be easy. I had a number of hurdles in the way:

- Legal experimental trials no longer allowed healthy people to participate
- The only other option was to go underground, but I needed to find someone I could trust, and even when I did find that person,
- How do I convince such a person to be my guide, knowing that I would write about it?

To put it mildly, I was really looking forward to go on a trip. By this time, I had heard so many people share their experiences that I longed to have something of my own to compare. I was dying to find out if, as many folks had said, this would be a transforming encounter for me, or if it could bestow upon my atheistic self, some acknowledgment of the divinity. In truth, I was also a little bit scared of some of the psychological dirt it could dig up from my past.

My journey to finding the right guide would make me realize that in many instances, underground guides are very close to the above-ground ones. I got a few recommendations for the former from the latter and from then on it was referral after referral. My interviews led me to discover Leo Zeff, one of the first underground therapists who died in 1988. Before his death, Zeff had recorded interviews with his friend, Stolaroff, in which he detailed his dilemma when psychedelic drugs were cancelled. According to him, it only made sense because he could not bear to watch people suffer or live an aimless life when they could get healing and enlightenment. Zeff was also one of those who helped create the code of conduct document guiding the underground psychedelic practice.

When the ban on psychedelic research was lifted in the late 1990s, the work of underground guides like Zeff proved useful as foundations on which to build new research. As I would later learn, the underground guides, often erroneously considered as a scattered bunch doing whatever they liked, were actually a group of organized people who ran their practices in accordance to established rules. In 2010, there was even a website containing all these carefully crafted documents. This realization filled me with much confidence. Considering the step I was about to take, I was relieved to find out that my initial thoughts were wrong.

Unfortunately, I didn't get reassured by the guides I interviewed at first. There was the Romanian guide with a nonchalant disposition who scared me and the weird man who chose food off the menu by swinging his tie. But my choice of guide was not the only concern here. I was also worried for my heart. I had had a health scare the previous year and I wanted the 'okay' sign from my cardiologist before embarking on this journey. His only note of warning was MDMA. I was not to go near that. Eventually, I would go with Fritz, a German living in a secluded mountain of the American West. In spite of more than one issues that should have struck Fritz off my list, I liked him immediately and that was it. After giving me a run-down of what my 3-day stay would entail and what I needed to do to ensure optimum experience, we were good to go.

My first day involved going into a trance by simply doing a breathing routine. I had the most exciting experience I had had in a while and actually felt myself let go. I surrendered to visions of myself expertly riding a horse. Fritz said my experience that first day was a good indication of how I would accept LSD. That night however, I experienced another heart scare that left me unsure as to whether or not I would continue the program. After a restless night of internal deliberation however, I was resolved to do exactly all I had planned on this journey. I however agreed with Fritz for an initial lesser dosage.

My LSD journey was vivid and interestingly filled most with images of my family. I felt a part of all the things I was experiencing and emotions I would not give much thought to on an average day gripped me with such a force that I shed tears. Fritz would later tell me I had voiced some resolutions while in that state; words that I would ordinarily consider weak and unnecessary. It was an enlightening experience indeed, but it was no encounter with God and neither did I lose the power to direct my consciousness. For a couple of days after this, I would exhibit effects of the journey. I was more relaxed and at peace with everything and everyone around me. Yes, I felt let down when this glow did not last, but my experience with LSD had instilled in me enough confidence to approach the next stage.

I chose Mary as my guide on the Psilocybin journey. She exuded a confidence and compassion that I found reassuring.

And I needed all the reassurance I could get with the size of psilocybin mushroom I was required to chew. It wasn't the prettiest sight and the taste was not much better, but Mary offered me chocolate, and the alternate bites I took of it helped me a lot. Prior to this, I had gone through a preparation ceremony which, according to my guide, was necessary to make me acceptable to the spirits. My psilocybin experience was different from the others; I didn't seem to have control over my stream of consciousness this time. I lay on that mattress, stuck in a videogame-like world where all I wanted was to get out. At one point during the journey, I had pause for a pee-break and when I looked at Mary, she was no longer Mary. She was Maria Sabina. I would later experience that ego-stripping that was common in many of the encounters I had interviewed. I witnessed the dissolving of myself yet felt totally at peace.

On my second pee-break, I made the mistake of looking into the mirror and saw a skull stare back at me. From then on, my journey turned dark, with ghosts of family members making an appearance one after the other. After an enlightening discussion with Mary, I would leave that place with a new perspective, a vivid understanding of my place in the world and how I was a part of everything else. It left me feeling light and at peace, and I wondered if this could be forever.

Unexpectedly, I came across another psychedelic, one which had not been the subject of extensive study as the rest. It had only been mentioned in the U.S in 1992 and even at that, there were no concrete facts or discoveries. But from the little I could glean about the Toad, it was way ahead of LSD and Psilocybin and I was genuinely doubtful if I could handle it. I decided to go for it. The reports were not false. The toad acted so fast that I did not remember inhaling it. I was blasted into a nothingness where everything that resembled self was blown to smithereens, yet I was aware. I wondered if that was what it felt like to be dead and strangely felt okay with that. The most astonishing thing happened after I felt my person slip back into place. I felt another person come out of me much in the same way I expect mothers feel their babies coming out of them. In my case, this person was my infant self whose face quickly morphed into my son's. I was further overwhelmed with a renewed sense of being and appreciation.

My encounter with the toad was mind-blowing and incomparable with all the journeys I had gone on before. For so long, I struggled to put it in an appropriate category-chemical reaction or mystical encounter? When I measured my experience using the questionnaire designed for the Hopkins and NYU volunteers, my score placed me in the mystical encounter category. Needless to say, I was disbelieving of this report because I didn't think my experience with the toad was what a mystical encounter should feel like. Despite my skepticism, I came away from these experiences a more sensitive man. My mind was enlarged and held the capacity for so much more; an openness that I had not known before. Events and things that I had hitherto overlooked bore a significance I did not try to overlook.

Maybe what we call the mystical is simply the result of an ego-free mind receiving what resides in the universe and as it appears, death loses some of its horror in that realm.

CHAPTER 5: THE NEUROSCIENCE Your Brain on Psychedelics

Key Notes:

- *New technologies have made it possible for researchers to investigate the link between the brain and psychedelic journeys*

- *Psilocybin and LSD act by attaching themselves to a receptor originally meant for serotonin*

- *Contrary to initial hypothesis, the brain records a decrease in activity during psychedelic journeys*

- *Psychedelic drugs act by shattering the system of order familiar to the human brain, making it possible to encounter new and psychedelic experiences*

- *To really grow, humans must embrace uncertainty and disregard their ego consciousness*

- *Children possess the ideal form of consciousness*

My journeys had such profound effects on me and I was curious to know how these substances had interacted with my brain and how that might provide valid explanations. What goes on in the brain from the time you ingest these substances to the time you realize your outlook on life has been changed, and long after the substance is worn off too.

The chemicals had one thing in common: they were tryptamines. It meant they were relatives of serotonin, a neurotransmitter located throughout the human body. But the relationship between these two groups was not clear until 1998 when Swiss researcher, Franz Vollenweider, proved that Psilocybin and LSD acted by attaching themselves to a receptor originally meant for serotonin. In an experiment, he demonstrated by blocking that particular receptor, resulting in psilocybin registering no effects.

Vollenweider's discovery, though helpful, still did not establish a link between the chemical and the consciousness it provoked. Fortunately, technology has come a long way from the early days of psychedelic research. There are imaging technologies that make it possible to compare brain activity measures with LSD and psilocybin presence, resulting in observable patterns from which we can make accurate deductions on the Brain-Mind link.

In 2009, Robin Carhart-Harris, David Nutt, and Amanda Feilding, joined forces to commence one of the most elaborate neuroscientific journeys using psychedelics. Carhart-Harris was testing the effect of psilocybin on people's brains by employing technologies like functional magnetic resonance imaging (fMRI) and magnetoencephalography (MEG) to scan changes in brain activity under the influence. The location of his program was David Nutt's lab and he was being funded by Feilding. Nutt was a renowned psychopharmacologist at the Centre for Psychiatry on the Hammersmith campus of Imperial College in West London.

Carhart-Harris was working on the assumption that psychedelics would occasion an increase in brain activity, but he got results to the contrary. The decreased brain activity was more prominent in the Default Mode Network (DMN), the part of the brain that lights up when we're doing stuff like mind-wandering, moral reasoning, self-reflection, and other similar processes. The farther the drop in a person's DMN, the more likely they were to report a dissolution of their ego. As it turned out, another researcher in America had similar results working with meditators. Decreased activity in the DMN was now linked to loss of self and a shattering of the familiar boundaries. This shattering is what results in the mystical experience of being at one with the world; having no self or identity outside the universe.

Carhart-Harris posits explanations for some of the commonly reported psychedelic experiences. He says that the brain's perceptive skills become less sharp during a psychedelic journey because of the attendant decreased activity. Still, on its way down, it struggles to create perception, resulting in distorted visions featuring similar images.

Our brains are highly efficient structures that save us time and energy by developing reliable codes of perception and responses. But here's the downside: all that order hinders us from accessing new experiences and unlocking greater consciousness. During a psychedelic journey, the DMN drops, making way for new connections to interact freely among the other sections of the brain. In no time, every sense of order programmed by the brain is dissolved, allowing for new experiences to swirl freely in the brain. This phenomenon is not without influence on the mental encounters of the sojourner. A good example is my psilocybin experience. My memory of Maria Sabina somehow interfered with my visual perception of Mary, my guide. This explanation also possibly applies to the many distortions that are a common feature of these journeys. As our brain slips from order into uncertainty, we are open to a myriad of mental states, some of which turn out to be transforming.

The modern science of psychedelics has provided explanations for a lot of phenomena, but it is yet to ascertain if the neural pathways formed during the psychedelic journey remains permanent or dissolves after the journey. The obvious explanation is embedded in the nature of learning as we know it. Without constant exercise, new neural circuits cannot be strengthened. In other words, the permanence of a transformation will depend on the individual's continued practice of the same. Carhart-Harris goes on to observe that even a temporary transformation has a lot of potential.

Entropy, that state of uncertainty, is not one many are comfortable with. We'd rather stick with the familiar patterns recognized by our brains than venture into the unknown. But without the latter, our consciousness is not expanded. I would come to identify two categories of mental states in myself. Feelings of gratitude, openness, and generosity provoked a sense of enlargement in myself. My ego is reduced and I am not occupied by my sense of self. On the other hand, I feel a sense of shrinking when I'm consumed with myself, experiencing fear or regret, or being obsessive. I know now that in the first state, DMN is off and uncertainty is high. In the second state, DMN is active and uncertainty is low.

In a supporting stand, developmental psychologist, Alison Gopnik proposes that the blissfully uncertain brain of a child, with its attendant consciousness, is the ideal. As adults however, we may be able to gain access only during psychedelic journeys. In her work, Gopnik contrasts the innocence and openness of child-like consciousness to the confident, orderly consciousness of adults that remained closed to exploration.

Gopnik and Carhart-Harris both believe in the possibilities of psychedelics. It can help infuse more uncertainty into the brains of healthy humans, jolting them out of familiar order and providing transforming experiences that may result in a better quality of life and greater productivity. Depression, Addiction, and Obsession-related illnesses can also be treated using psychedelics.

CHAPTER 6: THE TRIP TREATMENT Psychedelics in Psychotherapy

Key Notes:

- *Psychedelic research is kicking off and getting recognition again*
- *Studies have established its potency in erasing the fear of death in dying patients, as well as curing addiction and depression.*
- *At the center of the psychedelic experience is the loss of ego which is pivotal to the curative potential of psychedelics.*

For the longest time, one of the biggest challenges facing psychedelics is the reluctance of scientists to accept it as a valid therapeutic option. Not only can it not be tested scientifically, psychedelics contain a lot of subjectivities as well as claims of a mystical experience. These reasons account for the debates that have trailed psychedelics from their early days. Recently however, there have been efforts to resuscitate the study of psychedelics and incorporate them in psychotherapy. This comes at a time when mental disease is a nationwide problem that has so far defied various drugs and regimens. Psychotherapists, psychologists, and scientists generally seem to be showing more interest on the development of psychedelics. As one psychiatrist noted, much of the work being done now on psychedelics are building on what has been done, many of the works dating long before the 1960s.

Palliative care psychologist, Tony Bossis, and Psychiatrist, Stephen Ross were two men who were also hopeful about the incorporation of psychedelics into psychotherapy. Both men had been in charge of the NYU psilocybin cancer trials and were elated at the results. Many of their patients had reported a loss of fear. They had a new outlook to life that was profound.

There was the case of Patrick Mettes, who in 2010, was losing his battle with cancer. After coming across an article in the papers, he called NYU and signed up for the psilocybin trials. Patrick was first made to go through several sessions of therapy with Bossis, getting to know what he should expect from the journeys. Eventually, when time came for his psilocybin sessions, Patrick was guided by Bossis and another woman. He was advised to open up his mind to the new experiences, learning from everything.

Interestingly, it was not one of the experts on psychedelics who suggested administering the drugs to dying cancer patients. It was Aldous Huxley, and what he had in mind was for death to take on- to the dying- a more spiritual quality. His idea would be carried out on countless cancer patients in North America, Then in 1965, two years after Huxley's death, Sidney Cohen wrote a piece on the use of LSD in dying patients. He explained how an acid trip was capable of stripping the dying of their egos- the one thing that made death so frightful. Seven years later, Stanislav Grof and Bill Richards would share their experiences with patients who, after taking LSD, began to see death not as an expiration but as a transition to other realms.

When I did a review of Mettes' journey notes, all these claims seemed like child's play. He described an experience so gripping and intense and yes, transforming. He physically manifested the motions of putting to bed while on this journey; a sign that, he was convinced, indicated his rebirth. He left there without any fear for his cancer or even death. By the end of his session, he told his wife he had seen God's face. Interviewing other cancer patient volunteers would reveal that even though each had a peculiar experience, they shared some elements. All had encounters with death, and all said that they had gone through the process of rebirth. They all also came out of the experience without their fear of death. Even in the very last stages of Mettes' life, he had remained happy.

Disregarding queries on how true these accounts were, therapists and psychedelics experts- like Bossis and Roland Griffiths- had a surprisingly similar perspective summed up thus: if it was capable of helping their patients lose their fear of death, then it is of little consequence whether it is scientifically proven.

When, in 2016, the research findings of the NYU and Hopkins psilocybin cancer studies hit the newsstands, the support it got was a hopeful indication for psychedelic research. Even though the trials would have to be conducted on a larger scale for government to consider approval, this was a small win that had been a long time coming. Psychiatrist, Jeffrey Guss, would later explain the mechanism involved in Psilocybin's success. The natural human response to news of one's death is a series of "Why me?" questions. This is the ego at work, but with psilocybin, the ego is dissolved, giving way for a new, enlightened consciousness.

Patrick Mettes would go on to die a very conscious and peaceful death, radiating happiness up till his last breath. His wife attributes the peaceful man her husband had become in his last day to the psilocybin journeys he embarked on,

Interactions with people who had been cured of their addiction after their psilocybin sessions revealed a common thread: all of them talked about having a profound experience that changed their perspective of everything in the world. In the new levels of consciousness they attained, smoking was not such a big deal, and this made it possible for them to quit.

Matthew Johnson's 2009 psilocybin study with smokers yielded impressive results, but just as with the cancer trials, the more mystical a person's experience was, the better their therapeutic journey.

When Griffiths and Ross made their way to the FDA in 2017, they did not expect what they met. They had gone to seek approval for another psilocybin cancer trial when the FDA suggested looking into depression. They were thrilled! Something similar was happening in Europe with researchers and the European Medicines Agency (EMA). To a large extent, this was also inspired by the work of Robin Carhart-Harris who administered psilocybin to people suffering from treatment-resistant depression. Rosalind

Watts, who guided several of these psilocybin sessions noted that:

The volunteers portrayed their depression as being detached-from their younger selves, their values and principles, other people, and nature.

Their sessions made it possible for them to access troubling emotions that had been suppressed or buried by depression.

After their session, the volunteers all shared their experiences. They had to do with reconnection with the things and people they had lost touch with. They also had the strength and courage to face their darkest emotions, gaining freedom in the end.

Through all the accounts and literature on the psychedelic journey, the effect that stands out most significant and remedial is the loss of self. That one experience rings throughout, whether it is in treating mental illness or helping healthy people live a better life.

The End

CPSIA information can be obtained
at www.ICGtesting.com
Printed in the USA
LVHW040820250319
611720LV00002B/190

9 781950 284016